TOP 100 DRUGS

Pocket Reference Guide

ISBN: 1957426594
ISBN-13: 978-1957426594

ALBUTEROL

Brand Names

- ProAir RespiClick, ProAir Digihaler, Ventolin HFA, Proventil HFA

Pharmacologic Class

- Beta$_2$-agonist

Mechanism of Action

- Relaxes bronchial smooth muscle by binding to beta$_2$-adrenergic receptors.

Dosage Forms

- Inhalation (breath-actuated aerosol powder, solution), oral (tablet, syrup)

Common Uses

- Treatment or prevention of bronchospasm due to reversible obstructive airway disease; prevention of exercise-induced bronchospasm

Quick Facts

- HFA inhalers should be shaken well before each use. Prime prior to first use and when inhaler has not been used for more than 2 weeks by spraying into air 3 to 4 times.
- Mouthpiece of HFA inhalers should be cleaned at least once per week by removing the canister and running under warm water, then air-drying completely.
- Side effects: palpitations, tremors, dizziness, cough, nervousness

ALENDRONATE

Brand Names

- Fosamax, Binosto

Pharmacologic Class

- Bisphosphonate

Mechanism of Action

- Inhibits osteoclast-mediated bone resorption.

Dosage Forms

- Oral (tablet, effervescent tablet, solution)

Common Uses

- Treatment and prevention of osteoporosis; treatment of Paget's disease

Quick Facts

- Medication should be taken in the morning at least 30 minutes before the first food, beverage, and other medications of the day. Patient should stay upright for at least 30 minutes and until after eating to prevent esophageal irritation.
- Oral tablet should be taken with 6 to 8 oz. of plain water, and oral solution should be followed with at least 2 oz. of plain water.
- Side effects: abdominal pain, acid regurgitation, constipation, diarrhea, and esophagitis
- Less common side effects: osteonecrosis of the jaw, atypical femur fracture

ALLOPURINOL

Brand Names

- Zyloprim, Aloprim

Pharmacologic Class

- Xanthine oxidase inhibitor

Mechanism of Action

- Decreases the production of uric acid by inhibiting the action of xanthine oxidase.

Dosage Forms

- Oral (tablet), intravenous (powder for solution)

Common Uses

- Treatment of gout; prevention of tumor lysis syndrome and recurrent nephrolithiasis

Quick Facts

- Reduce dosage in renal impairment and titrate gradually.
- Take medication after meals to reduce gastric irritation.
- Patients should be counseled to immediately report a skin rash as it can develop into Stevens-Johnson syndrome or toxic epidermal necrolysis.
- Medication may take several weeks to have an effect.
- Side effects: diarrhea, nausea, precipitation of acute gout attacks

ALPRAZOLAM

Brand Name
- Xanax

Pharmacologic Class
- Benzodiazepine

Mechanism of Action
- Causes CNS depression by potentiating the effects of GABA (an inhibitory neurotransmitter).

Dosage Forms
- Oral (tablet, disintegrating tablet, solution)

Common Uses
- Treatment of anxiety disorders and panic disorder

Quick Facts
- DEA Schedule IV
- Black Box Warnings – Concomitant use with opioids increases risk of sedation, respiratory depression, coma, or death. Use of benzodiazepines has risks of abuse, misuse, addiction, physical dependence, and withdrawal reactions.
- Avoid alcohol, grapefruit, and grapefruit juice.
- Dose adjustment recommended in advanced liver disease.
- Side effects: drowsiness, dizziness, ataxia, lightheadedness

AMLODIPINE

Brand Names

- Norvasc, Katerzia

Pharmacologic Class

- Calcium channel blocker

Mechanism of Action

- Dihydropyridine CCB that blocks the transmembrane influx of calcium ions into vascular smooth muscle and cardiac muscle which results in increased peripheral arterial vasodilation and decreased peripheral vascular resistance.

Dosage Forms

- Oral (tablet, suspension)

Common Uses

- Treatment of chronic stable angina and vasospastic angina, hypertension

Quick Facts

- May worsen angina and increase the risk of MI after starting or increasing dose.
- Risk of peripheral edema can be minimized if medication is administered at bedtime and lower doses are used (2.5 or 5 mg/day).
- Side effects: peripheral edema, fatigue, reflex tachycardia, headache, flushing

AMOXICILLIN

Brand Names

- Amoxil, Moxatag

Pharmacologic Class

- Penicillin antibiotic

Mechanism of Action

- Inhibits bacterial cell wall synthesis by binding to one or more of the penicillin-binding proteins, which inhibits the final transpeptidation step of peptidoglycan synthesis in bacterial cell walls.

Dosage Forms

- Oral (tablet, capsule, powder for suspension, chewable tablet)

Common Uses

- Treatment of ear, nose, and throat infections (pharyngitis/tonsillitis, otitis media), genitourinary tract infections, *H. pylori* eradication, lower respiratory tract infections, skin and soft tissue infections, and sinusitis

Quick Facts

- Keep suspension refrigerated and discard after 14 days.
- Take at even intervals, preferably around the clock.
- Side effects: diarrhea, nausea, vomiting, rash

AMPHETAMINE-DEXTROAMPHETAMINE

Brand Names
- Adderall, Mydayis

Pharmacologic Class
- CNS stimulant

Mechanism of Action
- Blocks the reuptake of norepinephrine and dopamine in presynaptic nerve endings and increases their release into the extraneuronal space.

Dosage Forms
- Oral (tablet, capsule)

Common Uses
- Treatment of ADHD and narcolepsy

Quick Facts
- DEA Schedule II
- Black Box Warning – High potential for abuse and dependence. Assess the risk of abuse prior to prescribing, and monitor for signs of abuse and dependence while on therapy. Misuse may cause sudden death and serious cardiovascular adverse reactions.
- Use is contraindicated during or within 14 days of MAOI administration, including linezolid or methylene blue.
- Gradually increase dosing and avoid abrupt discontinuation to prevent withdrawal symptoms.
- Use with caution in patients with a history of seizures.
- Side effects: loss of appetite, weight loss, restlessness, nervousness, nausea, diarrhea

APIXABAN

Brand Name

- Eliquis

Pharmacologic Class

- Factor Xa inhibitor

Mechanism of Action

- Reversible and selective active site inhibitor of free and clot-bound factor Xa, resulting in decreased thrombin generation and thrombus formation.

Dosage Form

- Oral (tablet)

Common Uses

- Treatment and prophylaxis of DVT or PE; used to reduce the risk of stroke and systemic embolism in patients with nonvalvular atrial fibrillation (AF); prophylaxis of DVT in patients who have undergone hip or knee replacement surgery

Quick Facts

- Black Box Warnings – Premature discontinuation increases the risk of thrombotic events. To reduce risk consider coverage with another anticoagulant if apixaban is discontinued for a reason other than pathological bleeding or completion of therapy. Patients undergoing neuroaxial anesthesia or spinal puncture have an increased risk of epidural or spinal hematomas which could result in permanent paralysis.
- Dosage adjustment required in patients with renal impairment and nonvalvular atrial fibrillation (2.5 mg twice daily in patients with at least two of the following characteristics: age ≥ 80 years, body weight ≤ 60 kg, or serum creatinine ≥ 1.5 mg/dL).
- Side effects: hemorrhage, bruising, syncope, anemia

ARIPIPRAZOLE

Brand Names
- Abilify, Aristada

Pharmacologic Class
- Antipsychotic

Mechanism of Action
- May exert its effects through partial agonist activity at the dopamine D_2 and serotonin 5-HT_{1A} receptors, and antagonist activity at serotonin 5-HT_{2A} receptors.

Dosage Forms
- Oral (tablet, disintegrating tablet, solution), intramuscular (powder for suspension)

Common Uses
- Treatment of bipolar disorder, schizophrenia, major depressive disorder, Tourette's syndrome, and irritability associated with autistic disorder

Quick Facts
- Black Box Warnings – Elderly patients with dementia-related psychosis treated with antipsychotic drugs are at an increased risk of death. There is an increased risk of suicidal thoughts and behavior in children, adolescents, and young adults. Monitor all antidepressant-treated patients for clinical worsening and the emergence of suicidal thoughts and behaviors.
- May prolong the QT interval.
- Patients should be counseled to report signs of extrapyramidal symptoms, tardive dyskinesia (restlessness, tremor, stiffness, etc.), or neuroleptic malignant syndrome (sweating, fever, muscle rigidity).
- Monitor for hyperglycemia, dyslipidemia, weight gain.
- Side effects: anxiety, insomnia, nausea, headache

ATENOLOL

Brand Name

- Tenormin

Pharmacologic Class

- $Beta_1$-selective blocker

Mechanism of Action

- Binds to the $beta_1$-adrenergic receptors found in vascular smooth muscle and the heart, blocking the positive inotropic and chronotropic actions of endogenous catecholamines such as isoproterenol, norepinephrine, and epinephrine.

Dosage Form

- Oral (tablet)

Common Uses

- Treatment of hypertension, acute MI, and angina pectoris (chronic)

Quick Facts

- Black Box Warning – Avoid abrupt discontinuation in patients with coronary artery disease. Severe exacerbation of angina, MI, or ventricular arrhythmias have been reported in patients with angina.
- Contraindicated in patients with 2nd or 3rd degree AV block without a functioning pacemaker, bradycardia, cardiogenic shock, and overt heart failure.
- Medication can mask symptoms of hypoglycemia in diabetics.
- Side effects: bradycardia, hypotension, dizziness, fatigue

ATORVASTATIN

Brand Names

- Lipitor, Atorvaliq

Pharmacologic Class

- HMG-CoA reductase inhibitor

Mechanism of Action

- Inhibits HMG-CoA reductase, preventing the conversion of HMG-CoA to mevalonate (the rate-limiting step in cholesterol synthesis).

Dosage Forms

- Oral (tablet, suspension)

Common Uses

- Treatment of hyperlipidemia; prevention of atherosclerotic cardiovascular disease

Quick Facts

- CYP3A4 inhibitors can increase plasma concentration.
- Contraindicated in active liver disease.
- Avoid use in most pregnant patients (consider continuing therapy for patients at very high risk of heart attack or stroke). Avoid use when breastfeeding.
- Monitor LFTs at baseline and periodically thereafter.
- Limit alcohol intake and avoid grapefruit and grapefruit juice.
- Can be taken at any time of day.
- Side effects: diarrhea, arthralgia, myalgia, increased liver enzymes, UTIs, nasopharyngitis

AZITHROMYCIN (systemic)

Brand Names
- Zithromax, Zmax, Z-Pak, Tri-Pak

Pharmacologic Class
- Macrolide antibiotic

Mechanism of Action
- Binds to the 50S subunit of the bacterial ribosome, which inhibits RNA-dependent protein synthesis.

Dosage Forms
- Oral (tablet, powder for suspension, packet), intravenous (powder for solution)

Common Uses
- Treatment of community-acquired pneumonia, acute otitis media, COPD exacerbations, chlamydia, gonorrhea, and skin and soft tissue infections

Quick Facts
- Use with caution in patients with CrCl < 10 mL/min.
- Avoid concomitant use of aluminum or magnesium-containing antacids with tablet and immediate-release suspension.
- Do not refrigerate oral suspension.
- Patients should report symptoms of hepatotoxicity or severe diarrhea.
- Can prolong the QT interval.
- Side effects: diarrhea, nausea, vomiting, abdominal pain

BACLOFEN

Brand Names

- Lioresal, Gablofen, Ozobax, Fleqsuvy, Lyvispah

Pharmacologic Class

- Skeletal muscle relaxant

Mechanism of Action

- Believed to work at the spinal level to inhibit transmission of both monosynaptic and polysynaptic reflexes. Baclofen is a structural analog of GABA and binds to the GABA-B receptor, which decreases the release of excitatory neurotransmitters and substance P.

Dosage Forms

- Oral (tablet, solution, suspension, packet), intrathecal (solution)

Common Uses

- Treatment of spasticity, muscle spasm not due to rheumatic conditions, myoclonus, and muscle rigidity in multiple sclerosis and spinal cord injury or diseases

Quick Facts

- Avoid abrupt discontinuation to prevent withdrawal symptoms (sedation, somnolence and weakness, psychological symptoms).
- Avoid alcohol and other CNS depressants.
- Side effects: drowsiness, weakness, dizziness, confusion

BUDESONIDE-FORMOTEROL

Brand Name
- Symbicort

Pharmacologic Class
- Combination $beta_2$-agonist and corticosteroid

Mechanism of Action
- Budesonide inhibits inflammatory cells (mast cells, eosinophils, basophils, lymphocytes, macrophages, and neutrophils) and release of inflammatory mediators (histamine, eicosanoids, leukotrienes, and cytokines). Formoterol binds to $beta_2$-adrenergic receptors and increases the level of cAMP, which relaxes bronchial smooth muscle.

Dosage Form
- Inhalation (aerosol)

Common Uses
- Treatment of asthma and COPD

Quick Facts
- Prime inhaler prior to first use and when inhaler has not been used for more than 7 days by spraying into air 2 times. Shake inhaler well for 5 seconds before each use.
- Counsel patients to rinse mouth with water, without swallowing, after each use to prevent oral candidiasis.
- Side effects: headache, oral candidiasis, nasopharyngitis, upper or lower respiratory tract infection, allergic rhinitis, sinusitis

BUPROPION

Brand Names

- Wellbutrin SR, Wellbutrin XL, Aplenzin, Forfivo XL

Pharmacologic Class

- Dopamine-norepinephrine reuptake inhibitor

Mechanism of Action

- Inhibits the neuronal uptake of dopamine and norepinephrine and blocks nicotinic acetylcholinergic receptors.

Dosage Form

- Oral (tablet)

Common Uses

- Treatment of depression and seasonal affective disorder; smoking cessation

Quick Facts

- Black Box Warning – Increased risk of suicidal thoughts and behavior in children, adolescents, and young adults. Monitor all antidepressant-treated patients for worsening and the emergence of suicidal thoughts and behaviors.
- Contraindicated in patients with a seizure disorder, current or prior diagnosis of bulimia or anorexia nervosa, during or within 14 days of MAOI administration. Do not start bupropion in a patient receiving linezolid or IV methylene blue.
- Do not exceed 450 mg/day due to seizure risk.
- If used for smoking cessation, start 1 week before target quit date.
- Side effects: dry mouth, insomnia, tremors, headache

BUSPIRONE

Brand Name

- BuSpar

Pharmacologic Class

- Antianxiety agent

Mechanism of Action

- Majority of clinical effects believed to be due to its high affinity for serotonin 5-HT_{1A} receptors.

Dosage Form

- Oral (tablet)

Common Use

- Treatment of anxiety

Quick Facts

- May take 2 to 4 weeks for optimal effect.
- Avoid alcohol, grapefruit, and grapefruit juice while taking medication.
- Use is contraindicated during or within 14 days of MAOI administration. Do not start buspirone in a patient receiving linezolid or IV methylene blue.
- Use is not recommended in patients with severe hepatic or renal impairment.
- Can be taken with or without food but must be consistent.
- Side effects: nausea, dizziness, excitement, headache

CARVEDILOL

Brand Name
- Coreg

Pharmacologic Class
- $Beta_1/beta_2$-blocker and $alpha_1$-blocker

Mechanism of Action
- Blocks stimulation of $beta_1$ (myocardial) and $beta_2$ (pulmonary, vascular)-adrenergic receptors which reduces cardiac output, reduces exercise-induced tachycardia and/or isoproterenol-induced tachycardia, and reduces reflex orthostatic tachycardia. Blockade of $alpha_1$-adrenergic receptors causes vasodilation of blood vessels.

Dosage Forms
- Oral (tablet, capsule)

Common Uses
- Treatment of hypertension, heart failure, and impaired left ventricular dysfunction following MI

Quick Facts
- Contraindications include bronchial asthma or related bronchial spastic condition, 2nd or 3rd degree AV block, decompensated heart failure requiring IV inotropic therapy, and severe bradycardia.
- Avoid abrupt discontinuation in patients with coronary artery disease due to risk of exacerbation of angina, MI, or ventricular arrhythmias.
- Use with caution in patients with hepatic impairment.
- Take with food to decrease orthostatic hypotension.
- Side effects: hypotension, hyperglycemia, dizziness, fatigue

CELECOXIB

Brand Names
- Celebrex, Elyxub

Pharmacologic Class
- COX-2 inhibitor

Mechanism of Action
- Prevents the synthesis of prostaglandins by inhibiting the cyclooxygenase-2 (COX-2) enzyme.

Dosage Forms
- Oral (capsule, solution)

Common Uses
- Treatment of osteoarthritis, rheumatoid arthritis, ankylosing spondylitis, and acute pain

Quick Facts
- Black Box Warning – Increased risk of cardiovascular thrombotic events and GI bleeding, ulceration, and perforation. Contraindicated in the setting of coronary artery bypass graft surgery.
- Contraindicated in patients with an allergy to sulfonamides.
- Pregnant patients should avoid use starting at 30 weeks gestation due to the risk of premature closure of the ductus arteriosus.
- Avoid in patients with severe renal or hepatic impairment.
- Side effects: dyspepsia, headache, abdominal pain, upper respiratory tract infection, diarrhea

CEPHALEXIN

Brand Name

- Keflex

Pharmacologic Class

- Cephalosporin antibiotic (1st generation)

Mechanism of Action

- Inhibits bacterial cell wall synthesis by binding to one or more of the penicillin-binding proteins which inhibits the final transpeptidation step of peptidoglycan synthesis in bacterial cell walls.

Dosage Forms

- Oral (tablet, capsule, powder for suspension)

Common Uses

- Treatment of otitis media, respiratory tract infections, UTIs, skin and skin structure infections, and bone infections

Quick Facts

- Reduce dosage in renal impairment (CrCl < 30 mL/min).
- Use with caution in patients with a history of penicillin allergy.
- Keep suspension refrigerated. Discard unused portion 14 days after reconstitution.
- Side effects: diarrhea, abdominal pain, rash, hives

CHOLECALCIFEROL

Brand Name

- Delta D3

Pharmacologic Class

- Vitamin D analog

Mechanism of Action

- Cholecalciferol is converted to calcifediol in the liver, then to calcitriol in the kidney, which increases the absorption of calcium and phosphate in the intestines, the release of calcium from bone, and promotes the renal tubule reabsorption of calcium. Calcitriol also suppresses the synthesis of parathyroid hormone.

Dosage Forms

- Oral (tablet, capsule, solution, suspension)

Common Use

- Treatment of vitamin D deficiency

Quick Facts

- Patients should be counseled to report signs or symptoms of hypercalcemia, which include dry mouth, constipation, weakness, headache, arthralgia, nausea, and vomiting.
- Counsel patients to maintain adequate intake of calcium and to avoid additional vitamin D supplements.
- Side effects with high doses include hypercalcemia, nausea, constipation, loss of appetite

CITALOPRAM

Brand Name

- Celexa

Pharmacologic Class

- SSRI

Mechanism of Action

- Inhibits the reuptake of serotonin in presynaptic neurons of the CNS.

Dosage Forms

- Oral (tablet, capsule, solution)

Common Use

- Treatment of depression

Quick Facts

- Black Box Warning – Increased risk of suicidal thoughts and behavior in pediatric patients and young adults. Monitor all antidepressant-treated patients for clinical worsening and the emergence of suicidal thoughts and behaviors.
- Risk of dose-dependent QT interval prolongation. (Doses greater than 40 mg/day are not recommended.)
- May increase the risk of bleeding events. Concomitant use of aspirin, NSAIDs, warfarin and other anticoagulants can increase risk.
- Do not abruptly discontinue medication.
- Use is contraindicated during or within 14 days of MAOI administration. Do not start citalopram in a patient receiving linezolid or IV methylene blue.
- Patients should report symptoms of hyponatremia, which include headache, confusion, and weakness.
- Side effects: somnolence, insomnia, impotence, dry mouth, nausea

CLONAZEPAM

Brand Name
- Klonopin

Pharmacologic Class
- Benzodiazepine

Mechanism of Action
- Causes CNS depression by potentiating the effects of GABA (an inhibitory neurotransmitter).

Dosage Forms
- Oral (tablet, disintegrating tablet)

Common Uses
- Treatment of panic disorder and seizure disorders

Quick Facts
- DEA Schedule IV
- Black Box Warnings – Concomitant use with opioids increases risk of sedation, respiratory depression, coma, or death. Use of benzodiazepines has risks of abuse, misuse, addiction, physical dependence, and withdrawal reactions.
- Contraindicated in patients with significant liver disease and acute narrow-angle glaucoma.
- Side effects: drowsiness, dizziness, ataxia

CLONIDINE

Brand Names

- Catapres, Kapvay, Nexiclon XR

Pharmacologic Class

- Alpha$_2$-agonist

Mechanism of Action

- Stimulates alpha$_2$-adrenergic receptors in the brain, which reduces sympathetic outflow from the CNS to the heart, kidneys, and peripheral vasculature.

Dosage Forms

- Oral (tablet), transdermal (patch)

Common Uses

- Treatment of hypertension and ADHD (extended-release tablet)

Quick Facts

- Avoid abrupt discontinuation to prevent withdrawal symptoms, which include rebound hypertension, headache, tachycardia, nausea, and anxiety.
- Topical patches should be applied once weekly to a clean, hairless area of the upper outer arm or chest. If redness occurs a topical steroid may be applied to the area before application.
- Reduce dose in renal impairment.
- Side effects: dry mouth, drowsiness, headache, upper abdominal pain, impotence

CLOPIDOGREL

Brand Name
- Plavix

Pharmacologic Class
- $P2Y_{12}$ inhibitor

Mechanism of Action
- Inhibits the binding of ADP to its platelet $P2Y_{12}$ receptor which prevents activation of the GPIIb/IIIa complex and platelet aggregation.

Dosage Form
- Oral (tablet)

Common Uses
- Reduction of atherothrombotic events for patients with a history of recent MI, recent stroke, or established peripheral arterial disease; treatment of acute coronary syndrome

Quick Facts
- Black Box Warning – Effectiveness of medication will be diminished in patients that have reduced function of CYP2C19 (CYP2C19*2 and *3 alleles are nonfunctional).
- Rare cases of thrombotic thrombocytopenia purpura (TTP) have been reported. Symptoms include fever, fatigue, purplish bruises, and yellowing of the skin or eyes.
- Discontinue 5 days prior to elective surgery.
- Side effects: bleeding, bruising, rash, chest pain

CYCLOBENZAPRINE

Brand Names

- Flexeril, Amrix, Fexmid

Pharmacologic Class

- Skeletal muscle relaxant

Mechanism of Action

- Acts at the brain stem to reduce tonic somatic motor activity, influencing both gamma and alpha motor neurons leading to a reduction in muscle spasms.

Dosage Forms

- Oral (tablet, capsule)

Common Use

- Treatment of skeletal muscle spasm associated with acute, painful musculoskeletal conditions

Quick Facts

- Use is contraindicated during or within 14 days of MAOI administration. Other contraindications include hyperthyroidism, heart failure, arrhythmias, heart block or conduction disturbances, acute recovery phase of MI.
- Use with caution in patients with narrow-angle glaucoma, increased intraocular pressure or urinary frequency/hesitancy due to anticholinergic effects.
- Reduce dosing in patients with hepatic impairment.
- May enhance the effects of alcohol, barbiturates, and other CNS depressants.
- Side effects: drowsiness, dry mouth, headache, abdominal pain, constipation, diarrhea

DICLOFENAC (systemic and topical)

Brand Names

- Voltaren, Zorvolex, Flector

Pharmacologic Class

- NSAID

Mechanism of Action

- Prevents the synthesis of prostaglandins by inhibiting the cyclooxygenase-1 and cyclooxygenase-2 (COX-1 and 2) enzymes.

Dosage Forms

- Oral (tablet, capsule, packet), topical (gel, patch, solution)

Common Uses

- Treatment of osteoarthritis pain, acute pain, and actinic keratosis

Quick Facts

- Black Box Warnings – Increased risk of cardiovascular thrombotic events and GI bleeding, ulceration, and perforation. Contraindicated in the setting of coronary artery bypass graft surgery.
- Contraindicated in patients with a history of asthma, urticaria, or other allergic-type reactions after taking aspirin or other NSAIDs.
- Pregnant patients should avoid use starting at 30 weeks gestation due to the risk of premature closure of the ductus arteriosus.
- Avoid in patients with severe renal or hepatic impairment.
- Side effects: dyspepsia, nausea, headache, edema, diarrhea, constipation

DILTIAZEM

Brand Names

- Cardizem, Cartia XT, Dilacor XR, Tiazac

Pharmacologic Class

- Calcium channel blocker

Mechanism of Action

- Non-dihydropyridine CCB that blocks the transmembrane influx of calcium ions into vascular smooth muscle and cardiac muscle which results in increased peripheral arterial vasodilation and decreased peripheral vascular resistance. Also is a negative inotrope (decreased force) and negative chronotrope (decreased rate).

Dosage Forms

- Oral (tablet, capsule), intravenous (solution)

Common Uses

- Treatment of hypertension, atrial arrhythmia, paroxysmal supraventricular tachycardia, vasospastic angina, and chronic stable angina

Quick Facts

- Contraindications include hypotension (SBP < 90 mmHg), 2nd or 3rd degree AV block without a functioning pacemaker, and acute MI with pulmonary congestion on X-ray.
- Medication is both a substrate and inhibitor of CYP3A4.
- Do not abruptly discontinue medication.
- Side effects: peripheral edema, headache, dizziness, bradycardia

DOXYCYCLINE

Brand Names

- Vibramycin, Monodox, Doryx, Oracea

Pharmacologic Class

- Tetracycline antibiotic

Mechanism of Action

- Inhibits bacterial protein synthesis by binding to the 30S ribosomal subunit.

Dosage Forms

- Oral (tablet, capsule, powder for suspension, syrup), intravenous (powder for solution)

Common Uses

- Treatment of respiratory tract infections, anthrax, gonorrhea, acne, rosacea, and malaria prophylaxis

Quick Facts

- Medication should be administered with at least 8 oz. of water to prevent esophageal irritation or ulceration and with food to prevent gastric irritation. (Oracea should be administered on an empty stomach 1 hour before or 2 hours after meals.)
- Medication can cause photosensitivity. Patients should use sunscreen and avoid prolonged exposure to sunlight and tanning beds.
- Can cause permanent discoloration of teeth and should not be used during tooth development (last half of pregnancy, infancy, and children ≤ 8 years old).
- Avoid concomitant oral use with iron, bismuth subsalicylate, or antacids containing aluminum, calcium, or magnesium.
- Side effects: diarrhea, nausea, rash

DULAGLUTIDE

Brand Name

- Trulicity

Pharmacologic Class

- GLP-1 receptor agonist

Mechanism of Action

- Analog of incretin (glucagon-like peptide 1), which increases insulin secretion, decreases glucagon secretion, slows gastric emptying, and decreases food intake.

Dosage Form

- Subcutaneous (solution)

Common Uses

- Treatment of type 2 diabetes; risk reduction of major cardiovascular events in adults with type 2 diabetes and established cardiovascular disease or multiple cardiovascular risk factors

Quick Facts

- Black Box Warning – Causes an increased incidence of thyroid C-cell tumors in rats. The human relevance has not been determined. Dulaglutide is contraindicated in patients with a personal or family history of medullary thyroid carcinoma or in patients with multiple endocrine neoplasia syndrome type 2 (MEN 2).
- Refrigerate pens. If needed, each single-dose pen can be kept at room temperature for a total of 14 days.
- Administer once weekly without regard to meals.
- May cause pancreatitis.
- Side effects: nausea, vomiting, diarrhea, dyspepsia

DULOXETINE

Brand Name

- Cymbalta

Pharmacologic Class

- SNRI

Mechanism of Action

- Increases the synaptic concentration of serotonin and norepinephrine in the CNS by inhibiting their reuptake at presynaptic nerve terminals. Also weakly inhibits the reuptake of dopamine.

Dosage Form

- Oral (capsule)

Common Uses

- Treatment of depression, generalized anxiety disorder, fibromyalgia, chronic musculoskeletal pain, and diabetic peripheral neuropathy

Quick Facts

- Black Box Warning – Increased risk of suicidal thoughts and behavior in pediatric patients and young adults. Monitor all antidepressant-treated patients for clinical worsening and the emergence of suicidal thoughts and behaviors.
- Do not abruptly discontinue medication.
- Symptomatic improvement may take several weeks.
- Use is contraindicated during or within 14 days of MAOI administration, and allow 5 days after stopping duloxetine before starting an MAOI. Do not start duloxetine in a patient receiving linezolid or IV methylene blue.
- Monitor blood pressure regularly.
- Side effects: nausea, dry mouth, constipation, hypertension, sweating, sexual dysfunction in men

EMPAGLIFLOZIN

Brand Name

- Jardiance

Pharmacologic Class

- SGLT2 inhibitor

Mechanism of Action

- Inhibits the coupled reabsorption of sodium and glucose from the proximal renal tubules, thereby increasing renal glucose and sodium excretion.

Dosage Form

- Oral (tablet)

Common Uses

- Treatment of type 2 diabetes; risk reduction cardiovascular death in adults with type 2 diabetes and established cardiovascular disease; risk reduction of cardiovascular death and hospitalization for heart failure in adults with heart failure; to reduce the risk of sustained eGFR decline, end-stage kidney disease, cardiovascular death and hospitalization in adults with chronic kidney disease at risk of progression

Quick Facts

- Contraindicated in patients on dialysis.
- Reduce dose in renal impairment.
- Not recommended for use to improve glycemic control in patients with type 2 diabetes without established cardiovascular disease or cardiovascular risk factors with an eGFR < 30 mL/min/1.73 m^2.
- Stop 3 days before major surgery or procedures associated with prolonged fasting to decrease risk of ketoacidosis.
- Rare cases of Fournier's gangrene (necrotizing fasciitis of the perineum) have been reported.
- Side effects: Dyslipidemia, increased urination, urinary tract infection, genital fungal infection

ERGOCALCIFEROL

Brand Names
- Drisdol, Calciferol

Pharmacologic Class
- Vitamin D analog

Mechanism of Action
- Promotes calcium and phosphate absorption in the small intestine, the release of calcium and phosphate from bone, and renal tubule reabsorption of calcium and phosphate.

Dosage Forms
- Oral (tablet, capsule, solution)

Common Uses
- Treatment of vitamin D deficiency, rickets, hypoparathyroidism, and hypophosphatemia

Quick Facts
- Patients should be counseled to report signs or symptoms of hypercalcemia, which include dry mouth, constipation, weakness, headache, arthralgia, nausea, and vomiting.
- May be taken without regard to food, but it is better absorbed when taken with foods containing fat.
- Counsel patients to maintain adequate intake of calcium and to avoid additional vitamin D supplements.
- Side effects with high doses include hypercalcemia, nausea, constipation, loss of appetite

ESCITALOPRAM

Brand Name
- Lexapro

Pharmacologic Class
- SSRI

Mechanism of Action
- Inhibits the reuptake of serotonin in presynaptic neurons of the CNS.

Dosage Forms
- Oral (tablet, solution)

Common Uses
- Treatment of depression and generalized anxiety disorder

Quick Facts
- Black Box Warning – Increased risk of suicidal thoughts and behavior in pediatric patients and young adults. Monitor all antidepressant-treated patients for clinical worsening and the emergence of suicidal thoughts and behaviors.
- Risk of dose-dependent QT interval prolongation.
- May increase the risk of bleeding events. Concomitant use of aspirin, NSAIDs, warfarin and other anticoagulants can increase risk.
- Do not abruptly discontinue medication.
- Use is contraindicated during or within 14 days of MAOI administration. Do not start escitalopram in a patient receiving linezolid or IV methylene blue.
- Patients should report symptoms of hyponatremia, which include headache, confusion, and weakness.
- Side effects: somnolence, insomnia, impotence, dry mouth, nausea

ESTRADIOL

Brand Names

- Estrace, Climara, EstroGel, Vagifem, Vivelle-Dot

Pharmacologic Class

- Endocrine agent

Mechanism of Action

- Binds to nuclear receptors in estrogen-responsive tissues and regulates gene transcription and formation of mRNA. Also reduces the levels of luteinizing hormone and follicle-stimulating hormone secreted by the pituitary gland through a negative feedback mechanism.

Dosage Forms

- Oral (tablet), transdermal (gel, patch, solution), vaginal (ring, cream, tablet, capsule), intramuscular (oil)

Common Uses

- Treatment of vasomotor symptoms, vulvar and vaginal atrophy associated with menopause; prevention of postmenopausal osteoporosis; treatment of hypoestrogenism in females

Quick Facts

- Black Box Warnings – Estrogens increase the risk of endometrial cancer. Estrogens with or without progestins should not be used for the prevention of cardiovascular disease. Increased risks of MI, stroke, invasive breast cancer, pulmonary emboli, and DVT in postmenopausal women (50 to 79 years of age) using estrogens combined with progestins have been reported. An increased risk of developing probable dementia in postmenopausal women ≥ 65 years of age has been reported in women using estrogen alone or estrogen combined with progestins.
- Estrogens, with or without progestins, should be prescribed at the lowest effective doses and for the shortest duration possible.
- Side effects: cardiovascular or thromboembolic disorders, breast tenderness, headache, nausea

ETHINYL ESTRADIOL-NORETHINDRONE

Brand Names
- Loestrin, Nortrel, Ortho-Novum

Pharmacologic Class
- Oral contraceptive

Mechanism of Action
- Suppresses the production of luteinizing hormone and follicle-stimulating hormone, which prevents ovulation, and alters cervical mucus and the endometrial lining.

Dosage Form
- Oral (tablet)

Common Use
- Prevention of pregnancy

Quick Facts
- Black Box Warning – Cigarette smoking increases the risk of serious cardiovascular side effects from oral contraceptive use. Risk increases with age (> 35 years old) and heavy smoking (15 or more cigarettes per day).
- Contraindications include thromboembolic disorders, breast cancer, endometrial cancer, and severe hypertension.
- Medications that decrease the effectiveness of ethinyl estradiol-norethindrone include rifampin and St. John's wort.
- Take medication at the same time every day with no more than 24 hours between doses.
- Side effects: headache, nausea, breast tenderness, edema

ETHINYL ESTRADIOL-NORGESTIMATE

Brand Names

- Ortho Tri-Cyclen, Previfem

Pharmacologic Class

- Oral contraceptive

Mechanism of Action

- Suppresses the production of luteinizing hormone and follicle-stimulating hormone, which prevents ovulation, and alters cervical mucus and the endometrial lining.

Dosage Form

- Oral (tablet)

Common Use

- Prevention of pregnancy

Quick Facts

- Black Box Warning – Cigarette smoking increases the risk of serious cardiovascular side effects from oral contraceptive use. Risk increases with age (> 35 years old) and heavy smoking (15 or more cigarettes per day).
- Contraindications include thromboembolic disorders, breast cancer, and severe hypertension.
- Medications that decrease the effectiveness of ethinyl estradiol-norgestimate include rifampin and St. John's wort.
- Take medication at the same time every day.
- Side effects: headache, nausea, breast tenderness, edema

EZETIMIBE

Brand Name
- Zetia

Pharmacologic Class
- Antihyperlipidemic

Mechanism of Action
- Inhibits the absorption of cholesterol at the brush border of the small intestine, which decreases the delivery of cholesterol to the liver, reduces hepatic cholesterol stores, and increases the clearance of cholesterol from the blood.

Dosage Form
- Oral (tablet)

Common Use
- Treatment of hyperlipidemia

Quick Facts
- Patients also taking a bile acid sequestrant should take ezetimibe at least 2 hours before or 4 hours after the bile acid sequestrant.
- Patients should report symptoms of myopathy and rhabdomyolysis, which include muscle pain, tenderness, or weakness.
- Avoid use in moderate or severe hepatic impairment.
- Side effects: diarrhea, arthralgia, sinusitis, upper respiratory tract infection, pain in extremities

FAMOTIDINE

Brand Name

- Pepcid

Pharmacologic Class

- H_2 receptor antagonist

Mechanism of Action

- Inhibits histamine at H_2 receptors on gastric parietal cells, suppressing the concentration and volume of gastric acid secretion.

Dosage Forms

- Oral (tablet, powder for suspension), intravenous (solution)

Common Uses

- Treatment of GERD, erosive esophagitis, and peptic ulcer disease

Quick Facts

- Reduce dosage in renal impairment.
- Onset of action occurs within 1 hour and lasts approximately 10 to 12 hours.
- Discard unused suspension 30 days after reconstitution.
- Administer once daily (before bedtime) or twice daily (in the morning and before bedtime) as directed.
- May be used concomitantly with antacids.
- Side effects: diarrhea, constipation, headache, dizziness

FENOFIBRATE

Brand Names

- Tricor, Trilipix, Antara

Pharmacologic Class

- Fibric acid

Mechanism of Action

- Activates peroxisome proliferator activated receptor alpha (PPARα) which increases lipolysis, activates lipoprotein lipase, and reduces production of apoprotein C-III. This causes a lowering of VLDL and triglycerides and an increase in HDL.

Dosage Forms

- Oral (tablet, capsule)

Common Uses

- Treatment of hyperlipidemia and hypertriglyceridemia

Quick Facts

- Contraindicated in active liver disease, severe renal disease, gallbladder disease, and when breastfeeding.
- Avoid concomitant use with statins due to increased risk of myopathy and rhabdomyolysis.
- Patients should report symptoms of hepatitis, gallstones, pancreatitis, or a rash.
- Limit alcohol intake during therapy.
- Side effects: abdominal pain, dyspepsia, myopathy, rhinitis

FINASTERIDE

Brand Names
- Propecia, Proscar

Pharmacologic Class
- 5-alpha reductase inhibitor

Mechanism of Action
- Inhibits the type II isoform of the 5-alpha reductase enzyme, which blocks the conversion of testosterone to dihydrotestosterone.

Dosage Form
- Oral (tablet)

Common Uses
- Treatment of BPH and male pattern hair loss

Quick Facts
- Medication should not be handled by women who are or may be pregnant because absorption through the skin may harm a male fetus.
- New baseline PSA level should be established after 6 months of treatment and any increase should be evaluated.
- For treatment of BPH, 6 months of therapy may be necessary for maximal efficacy. For treatment of male pattern hair loss, 3 months of therapy may be necessary for clinical improvement.
- Side effects: decreased libido, impotence, breast tenderness

FLUOXETINE

Brand Names
- Prozac, Sarafem

Pharmacologic Class
- SSRI

Mechanism of Action
- Inhibits the reuptake of serotonin in presynaptic neurons of the CNS.

Dosage Forms
- Oral (tablet, capsule, solution)

Common Uses
- Treatment of depression, obsessive-compulsive disorder, panic disorder, premenstrual dysphoric disorder, and bulimia nervosa

Quick Facts
- Black Box Warning – Increased risk of suicidal thoughts and behavior in children, adolescents, and young adults. Monitor all antidepressant-treated patients for clinical worsening and the emergence of suicidal thoughts and behaviors.
- Risk of QT interval prolongation.
- Potent CYP2D6 inhibitor.
- May increase the risk of bleeding events. Concomitant use of aspirin, NSAIDs, warfarin and other anticoagulants can increase risk.
- Do not abruptly discontinue medication.
- Use is contraindicated during or within 14 days of MAOI administration. Allow 5 weeks after stopping fluoxetine before starting an MAOI. Do not start fluoxetine in a patient receiving linezolid or IV methylene blue.
- Patients should report symptoms of hyponatremia, including headache, confusion, weakness.
- Side effects: somnolence, insomnia, anxiety, dry mouth, nausea

FLUTICASONE PROPIONATE (nasal, inhalation)

Brand Names
- Flonase, Flovent, Arnuity Ellipta, ArmonAir Digihaler

Pharmacologic Class
- Corticosteroid

Mechanism of Action
- Inhibits inflammatory cells (mast cells, eosinophils, basophils, lymphocytes, macrophages, and neutrophils) and release of inflammatory mediators (histamine, eicosanoids, leukotrienes, and cytokines).

Dosage Forms
- Nasal (suspension), inhalation (aerosol, breath-actuated aerosol powder)

Common Uses
- Treatment of allergic and nonallergic rhinitis (nasal), asthma (inhalation)

Quick Facts
- Nasal spray may take several days of regular use for rhinitis symptoms to improve.
- Inhalation dosage forms may take 1 to 2 weeks of regular use for asthma symptoms to improve.
- When using nasal spray, shake gently before each use. Prime before first use and if not used for 7 or more days.
- When using HFA inhaler, shake gently before use. Prime inhaler before using for the first time, if the canister is dropped, or if it is not used for more than 7 days.
- Patients using inhalation dosage forms should rinse mouth with water, without swallowing, after each use to prevent oral candidiasis.
- Side effects for nasal spray: nasal burning or irritation, epistaxis
- Side effects for inhalation use: upper respiratory tract infection, oropharyngeal pain, sinusitis, headache

FLUTICASONE-SALMETEROL

Brand Names

- Advair Diskus, Advair HFA

Pharmacologic Class

- Combination beta$_2$-agonist and corticosteroid

Mechanism of Action

- Fluticasone inhibits inflammatory cells (mast cells, eosinophils, basophils, lymphocytes, macrophages, and neutrophils) and release of inflammatory mediators (histamine, eicosanoids, leukotrienes, and cytokines). Salmeterol binds to beta$_2$-adrenergic receptors and increases the level of cAMP, which relaxes bronchial smooth muscle.

Dosage Forms

- Inhalation (breath-actuated aerosol powder, aerosol)

Common Uses

- Treatment of asthma and COPD

Quick Facts

- When using the Diskus dry powder inhaler, do not exhale into the device, and use only in a level horizontal position. Discard device 1 month after it is removed from the foil pouch.
- When using the HFA inhaler, shake well for 5 seconds before each spray. Prime inhaler before using for the first time, if the canister is dropped, or if it is not used for more than 4 weeks.
- Counsel patients to rinse mouth with water, without swallowing, after each use to prevent oral candidiasis.
- Side effects: upper respiratory tract infection, nasopharynxgitis, oropharyngeal pain, sinusitis, headache

FOLIC ACID

Brand Name

- Folacin-800

Pharmacologic Class

- Vitamin

Mechanism of Action

- Folic acid is converted to tetrahydrofolic acid and methyltetrahydrofolate, which are required for the synthesis of thymidylate, purine nucleotides, and for normal erythropoiesis.

Dosage Forms

- Oral (tablet, capsule), injection solution (IM/IV)

Common Uses

- Treatment of megaloblastic and macrocytic anemias due to folate deficiency

Quick Facts

- Women planning a pregnancy and all women of child-bearing age should take folic acid (0.4 to 0.8 mg/day) to decrease the risk of neural tube defects.
- Doses greater than 0.1 mg/day may obscure pernicious anemia.
- Side effects: bitter or bad taste in mouth, loss of appetite, nausea, confusion, sleep pattern disturbance

FUROSEMIDE

Brand Name
- Lasix

Pharmacologic Class
- Loop diuretic

Mechanism of Action
- Inhibits sodium and chloride reabsorption in the proximal and distal tubules, as well as in the ascending loop of Henle.

Dosage Forms
- Oral (tablet, solution), intravenous (solution)

Common Uses
- Treatment of edema associated with heart failure, cirrhosis of the liver or renal disease, acute pulmonary edema, and hypertension

Quick Facts
- Black Box Warning – Furosemide is a potent diuretic which, if given in excessive amounts, can lead to profound diuresis with water and electrolyte depletion.
- Contraindicated in patients with anuria.
- Administer in the morning because of increased diuresis.
- Ototoxicity has been reported with rapid injection, severe renal impairment, higher than recommended doses, hypoproteinemia, or concomitant therapy with aminoglycosides, ethacrynic acid, or other ototoxic drugs.
- Infusion rate should not exceed 4 mg/min.
- Medication can cause electrolyte imbalances including hypokalemia, hyponatremia, hypocalcemia, hypomagnesemia, and hypochloremic alkalosis. Monitor periodically.
- Side effects: hyperuricemia, hyperglycemia, weakness, rash, photosensitivity

GABAPENTIN

Brand Names

- Neurontin, Gralise

Pharmacologic Class

- Anticonvulsant

Mechanism of Action

- Mechanism of action remains unknown. Gabapentin is structurally related to GABA, but it does not interact with GABA receptors or influence the degradation or uptake of GABA.

Dosage Forms

- Oral (tablet, capsule, solution)

Common Uses

- Treatment of postherpetic neuralgia; adjunctive therapy in the treatment of partial seizures (immediate release)

Quick Facts

- Reduce dosage in renal impairment.
- Patients should not use aluminum or magnesium-containing antacids for at least 2 hours before or after taking medication.
- Immediate-release dosage forms can be taken with or without food. Extended-release dosage form should be taken with evening meal.
- Avoid alcohol use.
- Avoid abrupt discontinuation in patients with seizure disorders.
- Side effects: drowsiness, dizziness, nystagmus, ataxia

GLIMEPIRIDE

Brand Name
- Amaryl

Pharmacologic Class
- Sulfonylurea

Mechanism of Action
- Stimulates insulin release from pancreatic beta cells.

Dosage Form
- Oral (tablet)

Common Use
- Treatment of type 2 diabetes

Quick Facts
- Take with breakfast or the first meal of the day.
- Avoid alcohol use.
- Concomitant use with a CYP2C9 inhibitor increases the risk of hypoglycemia.
- Patients should be counseled to monitor for signs of hypoglycemia (sweating, tremor, blurred vision, hunger, headache, etc.) and to always have a source of oral glucose available for treatment.
- Side effects: nausea, dizziness, asthenia, headache

GLIPIZIDE

Brand Name

- Glucotrol

Pharmacologic Class

- Sulfonylurea

Mechanism of Action

- Stimulates insulin release from pancreatic beta cells and may improve insulin sensitivity and decrease hepatic glucose production.

Dosage Form

- Oral (tablet)

Common Use

- Treatment of type 2 diabetes

Quick Facts

- Medication should be taken 30 minutes before a meal, preferably breakfast.
- Avoid alcohol use.
- Concomitant use with a CYP2C9 inhibitor increases the risk of hypoglycemia.
- Patients should be counseled to monitor for signs of hypoglycemia (sweating, tremor, blurred vision, hunger, headache, etc.) and to always have a source of oral glucose available for treatment.
- Side effects: diarrhea, nausea, dyspepsia, headache

HYDROCHLOROTHIAZIDE

Brand Names

- Microzide, HydroDiuril

Pharmacologic Class

- Thiazide diuretic

Mechanism of Action

- Inhibits sodium and chloride reabsorption in the renal distal convoluted tubule.

Dosage Forms

- Oral (tablet, capsule)

Common Uses

- Treatment of hypertension and edema

Quick Facts

- Contraindicated in patients with anuria or who have a hypersensitivity to sulfonamides.
- Administer in the morning to prevent nocturia.
- Medication can cause electrolyte imbalances including hypokalemia, hyponatremia, hypercalcemia, and hypomagnesemia. Monitor periodically.
- Use with caution in patients with gout. Medication can cause hyperuricemia.
- Use with caution in patients with diabetes. Medication can cause hyperglycemia.
- Usually ineffective in patients with a CrCl < 30 mL/min.
- Side effects: orthostatic hypotension, dizziness, weakness, photosensitivity, rash

HYDROCODONE-ACETAMINOPHEN

Brand Names

- Norco, Vicodin, Lortab

Pharmacologic Class

- Opioid analgesic combination

Mechanism of Action

- Hydrocodone binds to the mu opioid receptor, which reduces neuronal cell excitability and transmission of nociceptive impulses. Acetaminophen inhibits prostaglandin synthesis in the CNS and blocks pain impulse generation peripherally.

Dosage Forms

- Oral (tablet, solution)

Common Use

- Treatment of moderate to severe pain

Quick Facts

- DEA Schedule II
- Black Box Warnings – Serious, life-threatening, or fatal respiratory depression may occur. Concomitant use with benzodiazepines increases risk of sedation, respiratory depression, coma, or death. Concomitant use with CYP3A4 inhibitors, or discontinuation of CYP3A4 inducers, can result in a fatal overdose of hydrocodone. Prolonged use of hydrocodone-acetaminophen during pregnancy can result in neonatal opioid withdrawal syndrome. Acetaminophen has been associated with cases of acute liver failure. Use of hydrocodone-acetaminophen has risks of addiction, abuse, and misuse, which can lead to overdose and death.
- Patients should not exceed more than 4 grams of acetaminophen in a 24-hour period.
- Side effects: drowsiness, constipation, dizziness, nausea, vomiting

HYDROXYZINE

Brand Names

- Atarax (hydroxyzine hydrochloride), Vistaril (hydroxyzine pamoate)

Pharmacologic Class

- H_1 antagonist

Mechanism of Action

- Antagonist at peripheral H_1 receptors. Also suppresses histamine activity in the subcortical region of the CNS.

Dosage Forms

- Hydroxyzine hydrochloride: oral (tablet, syrup), intramuscular (solution)
- Hydroxyzine pamoate: oral (capsule)

Common Uses

- Treatment of anxiety, pruritis, nausea, and vomiting (intramuscular dosage form)

Quick Facts

- Use with caution in patients with asthma, COPD, BPH, and glaucoma.
- Avoid alcohol and other CNS depressants while taking medication.
- May prolong the QT interval.
- Side effects: drowsiness, dry mouth, headache

IBUPROFEN

Brand Names

- Motrin, Advil

Pharmacologic Class

- NSAID

Mechanism of Action

- Prevents the synthesis of prostaglandins by inhibiting the cyclooxygenase-1 and cyclooxygenase-2 (COX-1 and 2) enzymes.

Dosage Forms

- Oral (tablet, chewable tablet, capsule, suspension), intravenous (solution)

Common Uses

- Treatment of mild to moderate pain, rheumatoid arthritis, osteoarthritis, fever, and dysmenorrhea

Quick Facts

- Black Box Warnings – Increased risk of cardiovascular thrombotic events and GI bleeding, ulceration, and perforation. Contraindicated in the setting of coronary artery bypass graft surgery.
- Contraindicated in patients with a history of asthma, urticaria, or other allergic-type reactions after taking aspirin or other NSAIDs.
- Pregnant patients should avoid use starting in the third trimester due to the risk of premature closure of the ductus arteriosus.
- Use with caution in patients with renal or hepatic impairment.
- Side effects: heartburn, nausea, edema, diarrhea, abdominal pain

INSULIN ASPART

Brand Names

- Novolog, Fiasp

Pharmacologic Class

- Insulin, rapid-acting

Mechanism of Action

- Binds to the insulin receptors on muscle and fat cells and lowers blood glucose by increasing the cellular uptake of glucose and simultaneously inhibiting the output of glucose from the liver.

Dosage Form

- Subcutaneous (solution)

Common Uses

- Treatment of type 1 and type 2 diabetes

Quick Facts

- Novolog should be administered 5 to 10 minutes before a meal. Fiasp should be administered at the start of a meal or 20 minutes after starting a meal.
- Refrigerate unopened vials, pens, and cartridges. In-use vials can be stored in the refrigerator or at room temperature and discarded 28 days after initial use. In-use pens and cartridges should be stored at room temperature and discarded 28 days after initial use.
- Rotate injection sites to prevent inflammation and lipodystrophy.
- Side effects: hypoglycemia, lipodystrophy, rash

INSULIN GLARGINE

Brand Names

- Lantus, Toujeo, Basaglar, Semglee

Pharmacologic Class

- Insulin, long-acting

Mechanism of Action

- Binds to the insulin receptors on muscle and fat cells and lowers blood glucose by increasing the cellular uptake of glucose and simultaneously inhibiting the output of glucose from the liver.

Dosage Form

- Subcutaneous (solution)

Common Uses

- Treatment of type 1 and type 2 diabetes

Quick Facts

- Administer once daily at the same time every day.
- Refrigerate unopened vials and pens of Lantus and Semglee. In-use vials can be stored in the refrigerator or at room temperature and discarded 28 days after initial use. In-use pens should be stored at room temperature and discarded 28 days after initial use.
- Refrigerate unopened pens of Basaglar. In-use pens should be stored at room temperature and discarded 28 days after initial use.
- Refrigerate unopened pens of Toujeo. In-use pens should be stored at room temperature and discarded 56 days after initial use.
- Do not dilute or mix with any other insulin or solution.
- Rotate injection sites to prevent inflammation and lipodystrophy.
- Side effects: hypoglycemia, lipodystrophy, rash

INSULIN LISPRO

Brand Names

- Humalog, Admelog, Lyumjev

Pharmacologic Class

- Insulin, rapid-acting

Mechanism of Action

- Binds to the insulin receptors on muscle and fat cells and lowers blood glucose by increasing the cellular uptake of glucose and simultaneously inhibiting the output of glucose from the liver.

Dosage Form

- Subcutaneous (solution)

Common Uses

- Treatment of type 1 and type 2 diabetes

Quick Facts

- Administer within 15 minutes before or immediately after a meal.
- Refrigerate unopened vials and pens. In-use vials can be stored in the refrigerator or at room temperature and discarded 28 days after initial use. In-use pens should be stored at room temperature and discarded 28 days after initial use.
- Rotate injection sites to prevent inflammation and lipodystrophy.
- Side effects: hypoglycemia, lipodystrophy, rash

LAMOTRIGINE

Brand Name

- Lamictal

Pharmacologic Class

- Anticonvulsant

Mechanism of Action

- Mechanism of action remains unknown. Lamotrigine may produce its anticonvulsant effect by blocking voltage-sensitive sodium channels, which stabilizes neuronal membranes and modulates presynaptic release of excitatory amino acids, glutamate, and aspartate.

Dosage Forms

- Oral (tablet, chewable tablet, disintegrating tablet)

Common Uses

- Treatment of epilepsy (partial seizures, generalized seizures of Lennox-Gastaut syndrome, primary generalized tonic-clonic seizures) and bipolar disorder

Quick Facts

- Black Box Warning – Life-threatening skin reactions including Stevens-Johnson syndrome and toxic epidermal necrolysis have occurred. Incidence is higher in pediatric patients than adults. Risk may be increased when coadministered with valproic acid, high starting doses, or rapid increases in dose.
- Valproic acid increases lamotrigine concentrations by more than two-fold. Estrogen-containing oral contraceptives decrease lamotrigine concentrations by approximately 50%.
- Patients should immediately report symptoms of aseptic meningitis, including headache, stiff neck, fever, nausea, and vomiting.
- Side effects: dizziness, headache, diplopia, ataxia

LATANOPROST

Brand Names

- Xalatan, Xelpros

Pharmacologic Class

- Prostaglandin analog

Mechanism of Action

- Decreases intraocular pressure by increasing the outflow of aqueous humor through the trabecular meshwork and uveoscleral pathway.

Dosage Forms

- Ophthalmic (solution, emulsion)

Common Uses

- Treatment of open-angle glaucoma and ocular hypertension

Quick Facts

- Remove contact lenses before instilling medication and allow at least 15 minutes before reinserting.
- Wait at least 5 minutes before administering other ophthalmic products.
- Store unopened bottle in refrigerator. Once opened, can be stored at room temperature for 6 weeks.
- Side effects: pigment changes to eyelids and eyelashes, increased brown pigmentation of the iris, growth of eyelashes, conjunctival hyperemia, ocular pruritis

LEVETIRACETAM

Brand Names

- Keppra, Elepsia XR, Roweepra, Spritam

Pharmacologic Class

- Anticonvulsant

Mechanism of Action

- Mechanism of action remains unknown. Anticonvulsant effect may be due to modulation of synaptic neurotransmitter release through binding to the synaptic vesicle protein SV2A in the brain.

Dosage Forms

- Oral (tablet, solution, tablet for suspension), intravenous (solution)

Common Use

- Treatment of epilepsy (partial seizure, adjunct therapy for tonic-clonic seizure and myoclonic seizure)

Quick Facts

- Patients should report new or worsening depression, suicidal thoughts or behavior, or unusual changes in mood or behavior.
- Use with caution in patients with renal impairment.
- Avoid abrupt discontinuation, as this may increase seizure frequency.
- Side effects: somnolence, dizziness, asthenia, infection

LEVOTHYROXINE

Brand Names

- Synthroid, Levoxyl, Levothroid, Tirosint, Unithroid

Pharmacologic Class

- Thyroid product

Mechanism of Action

- Levothyroxine is a synthetic form of thyroxine (T_4). T_4 is converted to its active metabolite, L-triiodothyronine (T_3). T_4 and T_3 exert their physiological actions through control of DNA transcription and protein synthesis. This results in an increased metabolic rate, decreased TSH production by the pituitary gland, and effects on lipid and carbohydrate metabolism.

Dosage Forms

- Oral (tablet, capsule, solution), intravenous (solution)

Common Uses

- Treatment of hypothyroidism, pituitary TSH suppression, and myxedema coma (injectable form)

Quick Facts

- Black Box Warning – Medication should not be used for the treatment of obesity or for weight loss. High doses may produce serious or life-threatening toxic effects.
- Administer in the morning, preferably on an empty stomach, 30 to 60 minutes before breakfast.
- Do not administer within 4 hours of calcium or iron-containing products or bile acid sequestrants.
- Pregnancy may require higher doses.
- Side effects if dose is too high: palpitations, sweating, weight loss

LISDEXAMFETAMINE

Brand Name
- Vyvanse

Pharmacologic Class
- CNS stimulant

Mechanism of Action
- Exact mechanism of lisdexamfetamine in ADHD and binge eating disorder is unknown. Lisdexamfetamine is a prodrug of dextroamphetamine, which blocks the reuptake of norepinephrine and dopamine in presynaptic nerve endings and increases their release into the extraneuronal space.

Dosage Forms
- Oral (capsule, chewable tablet)

Common Uses
- Treatment of ADHD and binge eating disorder

Quick Facts
- DEA Schedule II
- Black Box Warning – High potential for abuse and dependence. Assess the risk of abuse prior to prescribing, and monitor for signs of abuse and dependence while on therapy.
- Use is contraindicated during or within 14 days of MAOI administration, including linezolid or IV methylene blue.
- Gradually increase dosing and avoid abrupt discontinuation to prevent withdrawal symptoms.
- Side effects: loss of appetite, weight loss, dry mouth, nausea, diarrhea, anxiety

LISINOPRIL

Brand Names

- Prinivil, Zestril, Qbrelis

Pharmacologic Class

- ACE inhibitor

Mechanism of Action

- Inhibits the angiotensin converting enzyme (ACE), which prevents the conversion of angiotensin I to angiotensin II, a potent vasoconstrictor.

Dosage Forms

- Oral (tablet, solution)

Common Uses

- Treatment of hypertension, heart failure, and acute MI

Quick Facts

- Black Box Warning – Discontinue use as soon as possible if pregnancy is detected.
- Contraindicated in patients with a history of angioedema, concomitant use with aliskiren in diabetic patients, concomitant use with neprilysin inhibitor, or within 36 hours of switching to or from a neprilysin inhibitor.
- Use caution in patients with impaired renal function.
- Patients should avoid potassium supplements or salt substitutes containing potassium without first consulting healthcare provider.
- Side effects: cough, dizziness, headache, hyperkalemia, fatigue

LISINOPRIL-HYDROCHLOROTHIAZIDE

Brand Name

- Zestoretic

Pharmacologic Class

- Combination ACE inhibitor and thiazide diuretic

Mechanism of Action

- Lisinopril inhibits the angiotensin converting enzyme (ACE), which prevents the conversion of angiotensin I to angiotensin II, a potent vasoconstrictor. Hydrochlorothiazide inhibits sodium and chloride reabsorption in the renal distal convoluted tubule.

Dosage Form

- Oral (tablet)

Common Use

- Treatment of hypertension

Quick Facts

- Black Box Warning – Discontinue use as soon as possible if pregnancy is detected.
- Contraindicated in patients with anuria, hypersensitivity to sulfonamides, a history of angioedema, concomitant use with aliskiren in diabetic patients, concomitant use with neprilysin inhibitor, or within 36 hours of switching to or from a neprilysin inhibitor.
- Patients should avoid potassium supplements or salt substitutes containing potassium without first consulting healthcare provider.
- Side effects: cough, dizziness, headache, orthostatic hypotension, fatigue

LORAZEPAM

Brand Names
- Ativan, Loreev XR

Pharmacologic Class
- Benzodiazepine

Mechanism of Action
- Causes CNS depression by potentiating the effects of GABA (an inhibitory neurotransmitter).

Dosage Forms
- Oral (tablet, capsule, solution), injection solution (IM/IV)

Common Uses
- Treatment of anxiety disorders and status epilepticus (injection)

Quick Facts
- DEA Schedule IV
- Black Box Warnings – Concomitant use with opioids increases risk of sedation, respiratory depression, coma, or death. Use of benzodiazepines has risks of abuse, misuse, addiction, physical dependence, and withdrawal reactions.
- Avoid alcohol and other CNS depressants.
- Metabolized to inactive compounds, therefore it may be less harmful for elderly patients or patients with hepatic impairment.
- Side effects: drowsiness, dizziness, lightheadedness, ataxia

LOSARTAN

Brand Name
- Cozaar

Pharmacologic Class
- ARB

Mechanism of Action
- Blocks the binding of angiotensin II to the angiotensin II type-1 receptor on vascular smooth muscle, which prevents vasoconstriction and the secretion of aldosterone.

Dosage Form
- Oral (tablet)

Common Uses
- Treatment of hypertension and diabetic nephropathy; used to reduce the risk of stroke in patients with hypertension and left ventricular hypertrophy

Quick Facts
- Black Box Warning – Discontinue use as soon as possible if pregnancy is detected.
- Contraindicated with concomitant use with aliskiren in diabetic patients.
- NSAIDs may reduce antihypertensive effect and increase the risk of renal dysfunction.
- Patients should avoid potassium supplements or salt substitutes containing potassium without first consulting healthcare provider.
- Side effects: dizziness, cough, nasal congestion, upper respiratory tract infection

LOSARTAN-HYDROCHLOROTHIAZIDE

Brand Name

- Hyzaar

Pharmacologic Class

- Combination ARB and thiazide diuretic

Mechanism of Action

- Losartan blocks the binding of angiotensin II to the angiotensin II type-1 receptor on vascular smooth muscle, which prevents vasoconstriction and the secretion of aldosterone. Hydrochlorothiazide inhibits sodium and chloride reabsorption in the renal distal convoluted tubule.

Dosage Form

- Oral (tablet)

Common Uses

- Treatment of hypertension; used to reduce the risk of stroke in patients with hypertension and left ventricular hypertrophy

Quick Facts

- Black Box Warning – Discontinue use as soon as possible if pregnancy is detected.
- Contraindicated in patients with anuria, concomitant use with aliskiren in diabetic patients, and hypersensitivity to sulfonamides.
- Administer in the morning because of increased diuresis.
- Patients should avoid potassium supplements or salt substitutes containing potassium without first consulting healthcare provider.
- Side effects: dizziness, cough, upper respiratory tract infection, back pain

LOVASTATIN

Brand Name

- Altoprev

Pharmacologic Class

- HMG-CoA reductase inhibitor

Mechanism of Action

- Inhibits HMG-CoA reductase, preventing the conversion of HMG-CoA to mevalonate (the rate-limiting step in cholesterol synthesis).

Dosage Form

- Oral (tablet)

Common Uses

- Treatment of hyperlipidemia; prevention of atherosclerotic cardiovascular disease

Quick Facts

- Contraindicated with concomitant use of a strong CYP3A4 inhibitor. Also contraindicated in active liver disease.
- Avoid use in most pregnant patients (consider continuing therapy for patients at very high risk of heart attack or stroke). Avoid use when breastfeeding.
- Monitor LFTs at baseline and periodically thereafter.
- Limit alcohol intake and avoid grapefruit and grapefruit juice.
- Immediate-release tablet should be taken with evening meal. Extended-release tablet should be taken at bedtime.
- Side effects: diarrhea, constipation, increased liver enzymes, dyspepsia, arthralgia

MELOXICAM

Brand Names

- Mobic, Vivlodex

Pharmacologic Class

- NSAID

Mechanism of Action

- Prevents the synthesis of prostaglandins by inhibiting the cyclooxygenase-1 and cyclooxygenase-2 (COX-1 and 2) enzymes.

Dosage Forms

- Oral (tablet, disintegrating tablet, capsule, suspension)

Common Uses

- Treatment of osteoarthritis and rheumatoid arthritis (disintegrating tablet and suspension only)

Quick Facts

- Black Box Warnings – Increased risk of cardiovascular thrombotic events and GI bleeding, ulceration, and perforation. Contraindicated in the setting of coronary artery bypass graft surgery.
- Contraindicated in patients with a history of asthma, urticaria, or other allergic-type reactions after taking aspirin or other NSAIDs.
- Pregnant patients should avoid use starting at 30 weeks gestation due to the risk of premature closure of the ductus arteriosus.
- Use with caution in patients with renal or hepatic impairment.
- Side effects: dyspepsia, nausea, diarrhea, constipation, abdominal pain

METFORMIN

Brand Names

- Glucophage, Glumetza

Pharmacologic Class

- Biguanide

Mechanism of Action

- Decreases hepatic glucose production and intestinal absorption of glucose, and improves insulin sensitivity by increasing peripheral glucose uptake and utilization.

Dosage Forms

- Oral (tablet, solution, suspension)

Common Use

- Treatment of type 2 diabetes

Quick Facts

- Black Box Warning – Metformin-associated lactic acidosis has resulted in death, hypothermia, hypotension, and resistant bradyarrhythmias. Risk factors include renal or hepatic impairment, age ≥ 65, having a radiologic study with contrast, surgery and other procedures, hypoxic states, and excessive alcohol intake.
- Contraindicated in severe renal impairment (eGFR < 30 mL/min/1.73m^2) and acute or chronic metabolic acidosis, including diabetic ketoacidosis.
- Medication can decrease folate and vitamin B_{12} absorption. Patients may need supplementation.
- Take with a meal to decrease GI upset.
- Side effects: diarrhea, nausea, vomiting, unpleasant metallic taste

METHYLPHENIDATE

Brand Names

- Ritalin, Concerta, Metadate ER

Pharmacologic Class

- CNS stimulant

Mechanism of Action

- Believed to block the reuptake of norepinephrine and dopamine in presynaptic nerve endings.

Dosage Forms

- Oral (tablet, chewable tablet, capsule, solution, powder for suspension), transdermal (patch)

Common Uses

- Treatment of ADHD and narcolepsy

Quick Facts

- DEA Schedule II
- Black Box Warning – High potential for abuse and dependence. Assess the risk of abuse prior to prescribing, and monitor for signs of abuse and dependence while on therapy. Use with caution in patients with a history of drug dependence or alcoholism. Chronic abusive use can lead to marked tolerance and psychological dependence.
- Use is contraindicated during or within 14 days of MAOI administration.
- Gradually increase dosing and avoid abrupt discontinuation to prevent withdrawal symptoms.
- Maximum wear time for patch is 9 hours/day. Do not expose patch to external heat sources.
- Side effects: decreased appetite, weight loss, nausea, insomnia, headache

METOPROLOL

Brand Names

- Lopressor (metoprolol tartrate), Toprol XL (metoprolol succinate)

Pharmacologic Class

- $Beta_1$-selective blocker

Mechanism of Action

- Binds to the $beta_1$-adrenergic receptors found in vascular smooth muscle and the heart, blocking the positive inotropic and chronotropic actions of endogenous catecholamines such as isoproterenol, norepinephrine, and epinephrine.

Dosage Forms

- Tartrate: Oral (tablet, powder for solution), intravenous (solution)
- Succinate: Oral (tablet, capsule)

Common Uses

- Treatment of hypertension, angina pectoris (chronic), acute MI (tartrate), and congestive heart failure (succinate)

Quick Facts

- Black Box Warning – Avoid abrupt discontinuation in patients with coronary artery disease. Severe exacerbation of angina, MI, or ventricular arrhythmias have been reported.
- Contraindications include 2nd or 3rd degree AV block without a functioning pacemaker, bradycardia, cardiogenic shock, and overt heart failure.
- Medication can mask symptoms of hypoglycemia in diabetics.
- Take oral dosage forms with food to increase absorption.
- Side effects: bradycardia, hypotension, dizziness, fatigue

MONTELUKAST

Brand Name

- Singulair

Pharmacologic Class

- Leukotriene receptor antagonist

Mechanism of Action

- Binds to the cysteinyl leukotriene receptor type-1 receptors in the airway (including airway smooth muscle cells and airway macrophages), which prevents airway edema, smooth muscle contraction, and airway inflammation.

Dosage Forms

- Oral (tablet, chewable tablet, packet)

Common Uses

- Prophylaxis and chronic treatment of asthma; prophylaxis of exercise-induced asthma; treatment of seasonal and perennial allergic rhinitis

Quick Facts

- Black Box Warning – Serious neuropsychiatric events have been reported and include agitation, aggression, depression, sleep disturbances, suicidal thoughts and behavior (including suicide).
- Montelukast is not for the treatment of acute asthma attacks.
- Avoid concomitant use with aspirin or NSAIDs in aspirin-sensitive patients.
- Chewable tablets contain phenylalanine.
- Side effects: upper respiratory tract infection, fever, headache, cough, abdominal pain

NAPROXEN

Brand Name
- Naprosyn

Pharmacologic Class
- NSAID

Mechanism of Action
- Prevents the synthesis of prostaglandins by inhibiting the cyclooxygenase-1 and cyclooxygenase-2 (COX-1 and 2) enzymes.

Dosage Forms
- Oral (tablet, capsule, suspension)

Common Uses
- Treatment of fever, mild to moderate pain due to osteoarthritis, rheumatoid arthritis, gout, dysmenorrhea, bursitis, tendinitis, and ankylosing spondylitis

Quick Facts
- Black Box Warnings – Increased risk of cardiovascular thrombotic events and GI bleeding, ulceration, and perforation. Contraindicated in the setting of coronary artery bypass graft surgery.
- Contraindicated in patients with a history of asthma, urticaria, or other allergic-type reactions after taking aspirin or other NSAIDs.
- Pregnant patients should avoid use starting at 30 weeks gestation due to the risk of premature closure of the ductus arteriosus.
- Use with caution in patients with renal or hepatic impairment.
- Side effects: heartburn, constipation, abdominal pain, edema, tinnitus, headache

OMEPRAZOLE

Brand Name

- Prilosec

Pharmacologic Class

- PPI

Mechanism of Action

- Suppresses gastric acid secretion by inhibiting the H^+/K^+-ATPase pump in parietal cells, blocking the final step of acid production.

Dosage Forms

- Oral (tablet, capsule, packet)

Common Uses

- Treatment of GERD, erosive esophagitis, *H. pylori* eradication, peptic ulcer disease, and Zollinger-Ellison syndrome

Quick Facts

- Take at least 30 to 60 minutes before eating.
- Do not abruptly discontinue. Medication should be tapered to avoid acid rebound.
- Strong CYP2C19 inhibitor.
- Use with caution with other medications that require an acidic pH for absorption (itraconazole, ketoconazole, iron, etc.).
- Patients taking long-term should have adequate calcium and vitamin D intake. (Calcium citrate formulations are preferred.)
- Short-term side effects: headache, abdominal pain, diarrhea, constipation, nausea
- Long-term side effects: increased risk of osteoporosis or fracture, vitamin B_{12} deficiency, hypomagnesemia

ONDANSETRON

Brand Name
- Zofran

Pharmacologic Class
- 5-HT_3 receptor antagonist

Mechanism of Action
- 5-HT_3-receptor antagonist which blocks serotonin peripherally on vagal nerve terminals and in the chemoreceptor trigger zone of the CNS.

Dosage Forms
- Oral (tablet, disintegrating tablet), injection solution (IM/IV)

Common Uses
- Prevention of chemotherapy-induced, radiation-induced, and postoperative nausea and vomiting

Quick Facts
- May mask signs and symptoms of bowel obstruction following abdominal surgery or chemotherapy-induced nausea and vomiting.
- Serotonin syndrome may occur when medication is used by itself or concomitantly with other serotonergic medications.
- Do not remove disintegrating tablet or film from packaging until immediately before use.
- May cause QT prolongation.
- Side effects: headache, diarrhea, fatigue, constipation

OXYBUTYNIN

Brand Names

- Ditropan XL, Oxytrol, Gelnique

Pharmacologic Class

- Anticholinergic

Mechanism of Action

- Inhibits the muscarinic action of acetylcholine on smooth muscle, which causes bladder smooth muscle relaxation.

Dosage Forms

- Oral (tablet, syrup), transdermal (gel, patch)

Common Use

- Treatment of overactive bladder

Quick Facts

- Contraindicated in patients with uncontrolled narrow-angle glaucoma, urinary retention, or gastric retention.
- Medication may cause heat prostration when used in a hot environment due to decreased sweating.
- Increased drowsiness may occur with concomitant alcohol use.
- Transdermal forms cause less dry mouth and constipation than oral forms.
- Side effects: dry mouth, blurred vision, urinary retention, constipation

OXYCODONE

Brand Names

- OxyCONTIN, Roxicodone, Xtampza ER

Pharmacologic Class

- Opioid analgesic

Mechanism of Action

- Binds to the mu opioid receptor, which reduces neuronal cell excitability and transmission of nociceptive impulses.

Dosage Forms

- Oral (tablet, capsule, solution)

Common Use

- Treatment of moderate to severe pain

Quick Facts

- DEA Schedule II
- Black Box Warnings – Serious, life-threatening, or fatal respiratory depression may occur. Concomitant use with benzodiazepines increases risk of sedation, respiratory depression, coma, or death. Concomitant use with CYP3A4 inhibitors, or discontinuation of CYP3A4 inducers, can result in a fatal overdose of oxycodone. Prolonged use of oxycodone during pregnancy can result in neonatal opioid withdrawal syndrome. Use of oxycodone has risks of addiction, abuse, and misuse, which can lead to overdose and death.
- Extended-release oxycodone is for use only in opioid-tolerant patients for the management of persistent, moderate to severe chronic pain that requires continuous, around-the-clock opioid administration for an extended period of time.
- Do not break, chew, or crush long-acting forms.
- Side effects: somnolence, constipation, pruritis, nausea, dizziness

OXYCODONE-ACETAMINOPHEN

Brand Names

- Percocet, Endocet

Pharmacologic Class

- Opioid analgesic combination

Mechanism of Action

- Oxycodone binds to the mu opioid receptor, which reduces neuronal cell excitability and transmission of nociceptive impulses. Acetaminophen inhibits prostaglandin synthesis in the CNS and blocks pain impulse generation peripherally.

Dosage Forms

- Oral (tablet, solution)

Common Use

- Treatment of moderate to severe pain

Quick Facts

- DEA Schedule II
- Black Box Warnings – Serious, life-threatening, or fatal respiratory depression may occur. Concomitant use with benzodiazepines increases risk of sedation, respiratory depression, coma, or death. Concomitant use with CYP3A4 inhibitors, or discontinuation of CYP3A4 inducers, can result in a fatal overdose of oxycodone. Prolonged use of oxycodone-acetaminophen during pregnancy can result in neonatal opioid withdrawal syndrome. Acetaminophen has been associated with cases of acute liver failure. Use of oxycodone-acetaminophen has risks of addiction, abuse, and misuse, which can lead to overdose and death.
- Patients should not exceed more than 4 grams of acetaminophen in a 24-hour period.
- Side effects: somnolence, constipation, pruritis, nausea, dizziness

PANTOPRAZOLE

Brand Name

- Protonix

Pharmacologic Class

- PPI

Mechanism of Action

- Suppresses gastric acid secretion by inhibiting the H^+/K^+-ATPase pump in parietal cells, blocking the final step of acid production.

Dosage Forms

- Oral (tablet, packet), intravenous (powder for solution)

Common Uses

- Treatment of GERD, erosive esophagitis, and Zollinger-Ellison syndrome

Quick Facts

- Take at least 30 to 60 minutes before eating.
- Do not abruptly discontinue. Medication should be tapered to avoid acid rebound.
- Use with caution with other medications that require an acidic pH for absorption (itraconazole, ketoconazole, iron, etc.).
- Patients taking long-term should have adequate calcium and vitamin D intake (calcium citrate formulations will have improved absorption in basic pH).
- Short-term side effects: headache, dizziness, diarrhea, constipation, abdominal pain
- Long-term side effects: increased risk of osteoporosis or fracture, vitamin B_{12} deficiency, hypomagnesemia

PAROXETINE

Brand Name
- Paxil

Pharmacologic Class
- SSRI

Mechanism of Action
- Inhibits the reuptake of serotonin in presynaptic neurons of the CNS.

Dosage Forms
- Oral (tablet, capsule, suspension)

Common Uses
- Treatment of depression, obsessive-compulsive disorder, generalized anxiety disorder, panic disorder, premenstrual dysphoric disorder, post-traumatic stress disorder, and hot flashes due to menopause

Quick Facts
- Black Box Warning – Increased risk of suicidal thoughts and behavior in pediatric patients and young adults. Monitor all antidepressant-treated patients for clinical worsening and the emergence of suicidal thoughts and behaviors.
- Potent CYP2D6 inhibitor.
- Associated with more weight gain than other SSRIs.
- May increase the risk of bleeding events. Concomitant use of aspirin, NSAIDs, warfarin, and other anticoagulants can increase risk.
- Do not abruptly discontinue medication.
- Use is contraindicated during or within 14 days of MAOI administration. Do not start paroxetine in a patient receiving linezolid or IV methylene blue.
- Patients should report symptoms of hyponatremia, including headache, confusion, and weakness.
- Side effects: somnolence, insomnia, dry mouth, nausea

POTASSIUM CHLORIDE

Brand Names
- K-Dur, Klor-Con

Pharmacologic Class
- Electrolyte supplement

Mechanism of Action
- Potassium is the principal intracellular cation of most body tissues and is essential for several physiological processes, including the maintenance of intracellular tonicity, the transmission of nerve impulses, the contraction of cardiac, skeletal, and smooth muscle, and the maintenance of normal renal function.

Dosage Forms
- Oral (tablet, capsule, solution, powder for solution), intravenous (solution)

Common Uses
- Treatment and prevention of hypokalemia

Quick Facts
- Normal adult plasma concentration of potassium is 3.5 to 5 mEq/L.
- Administer oral forms with food and a full glass of water to prevent gastric irritation.
- Potassium must be diluted prior to parenteral administration and should not be given IV push.
- Concomitant use with potassium-sparing diuretics, aldosterone antagonists, ACEIs, or salt substitutes containing potassium may cause hyperkalemia.
- Slow release potassium tablets and capsules should be reserved for patients who cannot tolerate or have compliance problems with liquid or effervescent dosage forms due to the risk of intestinal and gastric ulceration and bleeding.
- Side effects: vomiting, flatulence, abdominal pain, diarrhea

PRAVASTATIN

Brand Name
- Pravachol

Pharmacologic Class
- HMG-CoA reductase inhibitor

Mechanism of Action
- Inhibits HMG-CoA reductase, preventing the conversion of HMG-CoA to mevalonate (the rate-limiting step in cholesterol synthesis).

Dosage Form
- Oral (tablet)

Common Uses
- Treatment of hyperlipidemia; prevention of atherosclerotic cardiovascular disease

Quick Facts
- CYP3A4 inhibitors can increase plasma concentration.
- Contraindicated in active liver disease.
- Avoid use in most pregnant patients (consider continuing therapy for patients at very high risk of heart attack or stroke). Avoid use when breastfeeding.
- Monitor LFTs at baseline and periodically thereafter.
- Patients taking cholestyramine or colestipol concomitantly should take pravastatin at least 1 hour before or 4 hours after these medications.
- Limit alcohol intake.
- Can be taken at any time of day.
- Side effects: diarrhea, arthralgia, myalgia, increased liver enzymes, upper respiratory tract infection

PREDNISONE

Brand Names

- Deltasone, Rayos

Pharmacologic Class

- Corticosteroid

Mechanism of Action

- Binds to cytoplasmic receptors in cells. The steroid-receptor complex then enters the nucleus of cells where it modifies transcription and thus the synthesis of proteins and enzymes involved with inflammation.

Dosage Forms

- Oral (tablet, solution)

Common Uses

- Treatment of various allergic and inflammatory diseases (endocrine disorders, respiratory diseases, rheumatic disorders, etc.)

Quick Facts

- Patients on long-term therapy should avoid live or live-attenuated vaccines due to drug-induced immunosuppression.
- Take with food to decrease GI upset.
- Contraindicated in patients with systemic fungal infections because the infections may be exacerbated.
- Taper dose to prevent withdrawal symptoms if used longer than 2 weeks.
- Short-term side effects: insomnia, stomach upset, fluid retention, increased appetite
- Long-term side effects: Cushing's syndrome, osteoporosis, muscle wasting, growth suppression in children

PREGABALIN

Brand Name

- Lyrica

Pharmacologic Class

- Anticonvulsant

Mechanism of Action

- Binds to the alpha$_2$-delta subunit of voltage-gated calcium channels in the CNS, reducing the calcium-dependent release of excitatory neurotransmitters including glutamate, norepinephrine, serotonin, dopamine, substance P, and calcitonin gene-related peptide.

Dosage Forms

- Oral (tablet, capsule, solution)

Common Uses

- Treatment of fibromyalgia, neuropathic pain associated with diabetes or spinal cord injury, postherpetic neuralgia, and partial seizures

Quick Facts

- DEA Schedule V
- May cause peripheral edema. Use caution when using concomitantly with thiazolidinediones.
- May cause myopathy. Patients should report muscle pain, tenderness, or weakness.
- Avoid abrupt discontinuation. Taper gradually over a minimum of 1 week.
- Avoid alcohol and other CNS depressants.
- Side effects: weight gain, blurred vision, dry mouth, constipation, somnolence

PROPRANOLOL

Brand Names

- Inderal XL/LA, InnoPran XL

Pharmacologic Class

- Beta$_1$/beta$_2$-blocker

Mechanism of Action

- Blocks stimulation of beta$_1$ (myocardial) and beta$_2$ (pulmonary, vascular)-adrenergic receptors which reduces cardiac output, reduces exercise-induced tachycardia and/or isoproterenol-induced tachycardia, and reduces reflex orthostatic tachycardia.

Dosage Forms

- Oral (tablet, capsule, solution), intravenous (solution)

Common Uses

- Treatment of hypertension, angina pectoris (chronic), essential tremor, migraine prevention, and MI (early treatment and secondary prevention)

Quick Facts

- Avoid abrupt discontinuation in patients with coronary artery disease. Severe exacerbation of angina, MI, or ventricular arrhythmias have been reported.
- Contraindications include bronchial asthma, 2nd or 3rd degree AV block without a functioning pacemaker, cardiogenic shock, and severe sinus bradycardia.
- Infuse IV form at a rate of 1 mg/minute.
- Extended-release capsules can be taken with or without food but must be consistent. Immediate-release tablets should be taken with food.
- Side effects: diarrhea, dizziness, vomiting, fatigue

QUETIAPINE

Brand Name

- Seroquel

Pharmacologic Class

- Antipsychotic

Mechanism of Action

- Blocks dopamine D_2 and serotonin 5-HT_{2A} receptors. Also blocks histamine H_1 and alpha$_1$- and alpha$_2$-adrenergic receptors.

Dosage Form

- Oral (tablet)

Common Uses

- Treatment of bipolar disorder, major depressive disorder, and schizophrenia

Quick Facts

- Black Box Warnings – Elderly patients with dementia-related psychosis treated with antipsychotic drugs are at an increased risk of death. There is an increased risk of suicidal thoughts and behavior in children, adolescents, and young adults. Monitor all antidepressant-treated patients for clinical worsening and the emergence of suicidal thoughts and behaviors.
- Can prolong the QT interval.
- Patients should be counseled to report signs of extrapyramidal symptoms (restlessness, tremor, stiffness, etc.) or neuroleptic malignant syndrome (sweating, fever, muscle rigidity, etc.).
- Monitor for hyperglycemia, dyslipidemia, and weight gain.
- An eye exam for cataracts is recommended when beginning therapy and every 6 months thereafter.
- Side effects: somnolence, orthostatic hypotension, constipation, dizziness, dry mouth

RIVAROXABAN

Brand Name

- Xarelto

Pharmacologic Class

- Factor Xa inhibitor

Mechanism of Action

- Competitively inhibits free and clot-bound factor Xa, resulting in decreased thrombin generation and thrombus formation.

Dosage Forms

- Oral (tablet, suspension)

Common Uses

- Treatment and prophylaxis of DVT or PE; used to reduce the risk of stroke and systemic embolism in patients with nonvalvular atrial fibrillation (AF), and used to reduce the risk of major cardiovascular events in patients with chronic coronary artery disease or peripheral artery disease; prophylaxis of DVT in patients who have undergone hip or knee replacement surgery, and prophylaxis of venous thromboembolism (VTE) in acutely ill medical patients

Quick Facts

- Black Box Warnings – Premature discontinuation increases the risk of thrombotic events. To reduce risk consider coverage with another anticoagulant if rivaroxaban is discontinued for a reason other than pathological bleeding or completion of therapy. Patients undergoing neuroaxial anesthesia or spinal puncture have an increased risk of epidural or spinal hematomas which could result in permanent paralysis.
- 15 and 20 mg tablets should be taken with food.
- Side effects: bleeding, syncope, pruritis, muscle spasms, extremity pain

ROSUVASTATIN

Brand Names
- Crestor, Ezallor

Pharmacologic Class
- HMG-CoA reductase inhibitor

Mechanism of Action
- Inhibits HMG-CoA reductase, preventing the conversion of HMG-CoA to mevalonate (the rate-limiting step in cholesterol synthesis).

Dosage Forms
- Oral (tablet, capsule)

Common Uses
- Treatment of hyperlipidemia; prevention of atherosclerotic cardiovascular disease

Quick Facts
- CYP3A4 inhibitors can increase plasma concentration.
- Contraindicated in active liver disease.
- Avoid use in most pregnant patients (consider continuing therapy for patients at very high risk of heart attack or stroke). Avoid use when breastfeeding.
- Monitor LFTs at baseline and periodically thereafter.
- Limit alcohol intake.
- Patients should not use aluminum or magnesium-containing antacids for at least 2 hours after taking medication.
- Can be taken at any time of day.
- Side effects: abdominal pain, myalgia, nausea, constipation

SEMAGLUTIDE

Brand Names

- Ozempic, Rybelsus, Wegovy

Pharmacologic Class

- GLP-1 receptor agonist

Mechanism of Action

- Analog of incretin (glucagon-like peptide 1), which increases insulin secretion, decreases glucagon secretion, slows gastric emptying, and decreases food intake.

Dosage Forms

- Oral (tablet), subcutaneous (solution)

Common Uses

- Treatment of type 2 diabetes (Ozempic, Rybelsus); risk reduction of major cardiovascular events in adults with type 2 diabetes and established cardiovascular disease (Ozempic); weight management, chronic (Wegovy)

Quick Facts

- Black Box Warning – Causes an increased incidence of thyroid C-cell tumors in rats. The human relevance has not been determined. Semaglutide is contraindicated in patients with a personal or family history of medullary thyroid carcinoma or in patients with multiple endocrine neoplasia syndrome type 2 (MEN 2).
- Refrigerate unopened pens. In-use Ozempic pens can be stored in the refrigerator or at room temperature for up to 56 days. In-use Wegovy pens should be refrigerated but can be stored at room temperature if needed for up to 28 days.
- Store tablets in original bottle to protect from moisture.
- May cause pancreatitis.
- Side effects: Abdominal pain, nausea, vomiting, diarrhea

SERTRALINE

Brand Name
- Zoloft

Pharmacologic Class
- SSRI

Mechanism of Action
- Inhibits the reuptake of serotonin in presynaptic neurons of the CNS.

Dosage Forms
- Oral (tablet, capsule, solution)

Common Uses
- Treatment of depression, obsessive-compulsive disorder, panic disorder, post-traumatic stress disorder, social anxiety disorder, and premenstrual dysphoric disorder

Quick Facts
- Black Box Warning – Increased risk of suicidal thoughts and behavior in pediatric patients and young adults. Monitor all antidepressant-treated patients for clinical worsening and the emergence of suicidal thoughts and behaviors.
- Risk of QT interval prolongation.
- May increase the risk of bleeding events. Concomitant use of aspirin, NSAIDs, warfarin, and other anticoagulants can increase risk.
- Do not abruptly discontinue medication.
- Use is contraindicated during or within 14 days of MAOI administration, including linezolid or IV methylene blue.
- Patients should report symptoms of hyponatremia, including headache, confusion, and weakness.
- Side effects: somnolence, insomnia, headache, dyspepsia, nausea

SIMVASTATIN

Brand Names
- Zocor, FloLipid

Pharmacologic Class
- HMG-CoA reductase inhibitor

Mechanism of Action
- Inhibits HMG-CoA reductase, preventing the conversion of HMG-CoA to mevalonate (the rate-limiting step in cholesterol synthesis).

Dosage Forms
- Oral (tablet, suspension)

Common Uses
- Treatment of hyperlipidemia; prevention of atherosclerotic cardiovascular disease

Quick Facts
- Contraindicated with concomitant use of a strong CYP3A4 inhibitor. Also contraindicated in active liver disease.
- Avoid use in most pregnant patients (consider continuing therapy for patients at very high risk of heart attack or stroke). Avoid use when breastfeeding.
- Monitor LFTs at baseline and periodically thereafter.
- Limit alcohol intake and avoid grapefruit and grapefruit juice.
- The 80 mg dose should only be used in patients who have already been taking simvastatin for 12 months without signs of muscle toxicity.
- Take in the evening for maximal efficacy.
- Side effects: constipation, myalgia, abdominal pain, upper respiratory tract infection

SITAGLIPTIN

Brand Name

- Januvia

Pharmacologic Class

- DPP-4 inhibitor

Mechanism of Action

- Prevents the dipeptidyl peptidase-4 (DPP-4) enzyme from degrading the incretin hormones glucagon-like peptide-1 (GLP-1) and glucose-dependent insulinotropic polypeptide (GIP). These hormones increase insulin release and decrease glucagon levels.

Dosage Form

- Oral (tablet)

Common Use

- Treatment of type 2 diabetes

Quick Facts

- Reduce dosage in renal impairment (eGFR < 45 mL/min/1.73m^2).
- Patients should be counseled to report symptoms of congestive heart failure, acute pancreatitis, and bullous pemphigoid.
- Side effects: upper respiratory tract infection, nasopharyngitis, headache

SPIRONOLACTONE

Brand Names
- Aldactone, CaroSpir

Pharmacologic Class
- Aldosterone receptor antagonist and potassium-sparing diuretic

Mechanism of Action
- Competes with aldosterone for receptor sites in the distal convoluted tubules to increase sodium, chloride, and water excretion, and decrease the excretion of potassium.

Dosage Forms
- Oral (tablet, suspension)

Common Uses
- Treatment of heart failure with reduced ejection fraction, hypertension, edema associated with hepatic cirrhosis or nephrotic syndrome, and primary hyperaldosteronism (tablets only)

Quick Facts
- Contraindicated in patients with hyperkalemia, Addison's disease, and concomitant use of eplerenone.
- Administer in the morning because of increased diuresis.
- Medication can cause electrolyte imbalances, including hyperkalemia, hyponatremia, hypocalcemia, hypomagnesemia, and hypochloremic alkalosis. Monitor potassium levels within 1 week of initiation or titration, then monitor potassium and other electrolytes periodically thereafter.
- Patients should avoid potassium supplements and foods containing high levels of potassium, including salt substitutes.
- Can be taken with or without food but must be consistent.
- Side effects: gynecomastia, menstrual changes, hirsutism, diarrhea, nausea

TAMSULOSIN

Brand Name
- Flomax

Pharmacologic Class
- Alpha$_1$-blocker

Mechanism of Action
- Antagonist of alpha$_{1A}$-adrenergic receptors in the prostate, which relaxes the smooth muscle of the prostate and bladder neck.

Dosage Form
- Oral (capsule)

Common Use
- Treatment of BPH

Quick Facts
- Administer medication 30 minutes after the same meal each day.
- Medication may cause orthostatic hypotension, especially with first dose or a dose increase. Patients should be counseled to rise slowly from a sitting or lying position.
- Patients undergoing cataract or glaucoma surgery should inform the surgeon that they take or have taken tamsulosin due to the risk of intraoperative floppy iris syndrome (IFIS).
- Side effects: headache, dizziness, back pain, asthenia

TIZANIDINE

Brand Name

- Zanaflex

Pharmacologic Class

- Skeletal muscle relaxant

Mechanism of Action

- Agonist at alpha$_2$-adrenergic receptors and is thought to reduce spasticity by increasing presynaptic inhibition of motor neurons.

Dosage Forms

- Oral (tablet, capsule)

Common Use

- Treatment of spasticity

Quick Facts

- Tablets and capsules are bioequivalent under fasted conditions, but not under fed conditions. When taken with food, plasma concentrations of the tablet form are increased and the plasma concentrations of the capsule form are decreased.
- Monitor liver function at baseline and 1 month after maximum dose is achieved, or if hepatic injury is suspected.
- Use with caution when taken concurrently with other CNS depressants.
- Avoid abrupt discontinuation of medication. Withdrawal, rebound hypertension, tachycardia, and hypertonia may occur.
- Avoid alcohol use.
- Side effects: drowsiness, dizziness, hypotension, dry mouth

TOPIRAMATE

Brand Names
- Topamax, Qudexy XR, Trokendi XR, Eprontia

Pharmacologic Class
- Anticonvulsant

Mechanism of Action
- Exact mechanism is unknown. Activity may be due to blocking voltage-dependent sodium channels, enhancing GABA-A activity, antagonizing AMPA/kainate glutamate receptors, and inhibiting carbonic anhydrase.

Dosage Forms
- Oral (tablet, capsule, solution)

Common Uses
- Treatment of epilepsy (partial seizure, tonic-clonic seizure, Lennox-Gastaut syndrome); migraine prophylaxis

Quick Facts
- Medication may cause metabolic acidosis. Monitor serum bicarbonate at baseline and periodically during therapy.
- Decreased sweating and hyperthermia may occur, especially in pediatric patients.
- Taking during pregnancy increases the risk of oral cleft birth defects.
- Stay well hydrated during therapy to reduce the risk of kidney stone formation.
- Side effects: weight loss, abnormal vision, memory or concentration difficulties, fatigue

TRAMADOL

Brand Names
- Ultram, ConZip, Qdolo

Pharmacologic Class
- Opioid analgesic

Mechanism of Action
- Binds to the mu opioid receptor, which reduces neuronal cell excitability and transmission of nociceptive impulses. Also inhibits the reuptake of norepinephrine and serotonin, which activate descending pain inhibitory pathways.

Dosage Forms
- Oral (tablet, capsule, solution)

Common Use
- Treatment of moderate to severe pain

Quick Facts
- DEA Schedule IV
- Black Box Warnings – Serious, life-threatening, or fatal respiratory depression may occur. Concomitant use with benzodiazepines increases risk of sedation, respiratory depression, coma, or death. Concomitant use or discontinuation of CYP3A4 inducers, 3A4 inhibitors, or 2D6 inhibitors with tramadol requires careful consideration of the effects on tramadol and its active metabolite. Prolonged use of tramadol during pregnancy can result in neonatal opioid withdrawal syndrome. Contraindicated in children < 12 years of age and in children < 18 years of age following tonsillectomy and/or adenoidectomy. Use of tramadol has risks of addiction, abuse, and misuse, which can lead to overdose and death.
- Seizures have been reported even when taken within recommended dosage range. Risk increases with doses exceeding recommended range or with concomitant use with medications that decrease seizure threshold.
- Serotonin syndrome may occur, particularly with concomitant use of serotonergic medications.
- Side effects: pruritis, constipation, sweating, somnolence

TRAZODONE

Brand Names

- Desyrel, Oleptro

Pharmacologic Class

- SARI (Serotonin antagonist and reuptake inhibitor)

Mechanism of Action

- Inhibits the neuronal reuptake of serotonin and acts as an antagonist at 5-$HT_{2A/2C}$ serotonin receptors. Also blocks histamine and $alpha_1$-adrenergic receptors.

Dosage Form

- Oral (tablet)

Common Uses

- Treatment of insomnia and depression

Quick Facts

- Black Box Warning – Increased risk of suicidal thoughts and behavior in pediatric patients and young adults. Monitor all antidepressant-treated patients for clinical worsening and the emergence of suicidal thoughts and behaviors.
- Use is contraindicated during or within 14 days of MAOI administration. Do not start trazodone in a patient receiving linezolid or IV methylene blue.
- May cause QT prolongation.
- Grapefruit juice and CYP3A4 inhibitors can increase levels of trazodone.
- Immediate-release tablets should be taken after a meal or light snack. Extended-release tablets should be taken on an empty stomach.
- Side effects: drowsiness, orthostatic hypotension, syncope, priapism

VENLAFAXINE

Brand Name
- Effexor

Pharmacologic Class
- SNRI

Mechanism of Action
- Increases the synaptic concentration of serotonin and norepinephrine in the CNS by inhibiting their reuptake at presynaptic nerve terminals. Also weakly inhibits the reuptake of dopamine.

Dosage Forms
- Oral (tablet, capsule)

Common Uses
- Treatment of depression, generalized anxiety disorder, panic disorder, and social anxiety disorder

Quick Facts
- Black Box Warning – Increased risk of suicidal thoughts and behavior in pediatric patients and young adults. Monitor all antidepressant-treated patients for clinical worsening and the emergence of suicidal thoughts and behaviors.
- Do not abruptly discontinue medication.
- Symptomatic improvement may take several weeks.
- Use is contraindicated during or within 14 days of MAOI administration, and allow 7 days after stopping venlafaxine before starting an MAOI. Do not start venlafaxine in a patient receiving linezolid or IV methylene blue.
- Monitor blood pressure regularly.
- Side effects: nausea, dry mouth, constipation, hypertension, sweating, sexual dysfunction in men

WARFARIN

Brand Names
- Coumadin, Jantoven

Pharmacologic Class
- Anticoagulant

Mechanism of Action
- Blocks the function of the vitamin K epoxide reductase complex, which inhibits the synthesis of vitamin-K dependent clotting factors (II, VII, IX, and X) and proteins C and S.

Dosage Form
- Oral (tablet)

Common Uses
- Prophylaxis and treatment of venous thrombosis, arising pulmonary embolisms, and thromboembolic complications from atrial fibrillation or cardiac valve replacement; used to reduce the risk of death, recurrent MI, and thromboembolic events (e.g., stroke, systemic embolization) after MI

Quick Facts
- Black Box Warning – Warfarin can cause major or fatal bleeding. All treated patients should have regular INR monitoring. Drugs, dietary changes, and other factors affect INR levels. Instruct patients about prevention measures to minimize risk of bleeding and to report signs and symptoms of bleeding.
- Inhibitors and inducers of CYP2C9, 1A2, or 3A4 may affect warfarin levels.
- Patients should contact prescriber immediately if they have symptoms of purple toe syndrome or warfarin-induced skin necrosis.
- Dietary vitamin K must be consistent.
- Side effects: nausea, abdominal pain, rash, chills

ZOLPIDEM

Brand Names
- Ambien, Edluar, Intermezzo

Pharmacologic Class
- Hypnotic

Mechanism of Action
- Increases the activity of GABA by selective agonism at the benzodiazepine-1 receptor.

Dosage Forms
- Oral (tablet, capsule, sublingual tablet)

Common Use
- Treatment of insomnia

Quick Facts
- DEA Schedule IV
- Black Box Warning – Complex sleep behaviors including sleep-walking, sleep-driving, and engaging in other activities while not fully awake may occur. Discontinue medication immediately if a patient experiences a complex sleep behavior. Use is contraindicated in patients who have experienced these events.
- Administer medication immediately before bedtime. Do not take with or immediately following a meal, as it may delay onset.
- Avoid alcohol and other CNS depressants.
- Side effects in short-term trials: drowsiness, dizziness
- Side effects in long-term trials: dizziness, drugged feelings, lethargy

INDEX

I – L

M

N – O

P – Q

R – S

T – V

W – Z

Made in the USA
Monee, IL
13 September 2026

62976607R00059